Ketogenic Diet: Detox Diet:

Weight Loss for Beginners & Detox Cleanse to Heal the Inflammation, Lose Belly Fat & Increase Energy

Emma Rose

Ketogenic Diet Guide for Beginners

How to Achieve Rapid Weight Loss, Optimal Health & Unstoppable Energy with Ketogenic Diet Recipes

Emma Rose

Table Of Contents

Introduction

I want to thank you and congratulate you for purchasing the book, *"**Ketogenic Diet Guide for Beginners:** How to Achieve Rapid Weight Loss, Optimal Health & Unstoppable Energy with Ketogenic Diet Recipes"*.

This book contains proven steps and strategies on how to lose weight by following the ketogenic diet.

This diet has been around for decades, used in the clinical management of epilepsy. Over years of study, it has been found the ketosis is an effective way to lose stubborn fat. It is a very effective way burn the fats and keeps them off. the idea of burning fat by eating may seem incredulous to some. Read on and find out just how the ketogenic diet is done and how to do it properly. You also get to have a few sample recipes that work with the ketogenic diet. Eating for health and weight loss has never been so much fun.

Thanks again for purchasing this book, I hope you enjoy it! Please take some time to stop by and LIKE our Facebook page:

https://www.facebook.com/joypublishing

With gratitude,

Emma Rose

Chapter 1 What The Ketogenic Diet is All About

This is not a new diet. The ketogenic diet is actually a diet formulated decades ago as a part of the management of epilepsy. In recent years, it has been discovered that this same diet can help in reducing weight.

The ketogenic diet is one that places the body into a state of ketosis. In this state, the body relies on fat burning as a way to produce the energy it needs for various metabolic and homeostatic processes. Normally, the body relies on the conversion of carbohydrates into glucose as an energy source. This same process, however, also promotes weight gain. In response to the presence of glucose in the blood, the body releases insulin. This hormone is important because it allows glucose to enter the cells and be used as energy. Without insulin, glucose will remain in the blood, accumulate and cause hyperglycemia, a condition that can cause health problems if not managed quickly. At the same time that insulin allows glucose to enter cells, it also promotes some of the glucose to be stored by the body, which results in weight gain.

In ketosis, instead of using glucose, the body uses ketones. These are energy molecules released as a by-product of fat metabolism. By using ketones, the body does not have to release insulin. Therefore none of the ketones are stored that can add to weight. Any ketones that remain in the blood and not used by the body are excreted via the kidneys. Hence, by using ketones as energy source, the body is still able to function at optimum, and the excess are not stored as fats, unlike when glucose is used.

Is the ketogenic diet effective for weight loss?

Ketogenic diet is effective in losing weight because it limits the consumption of carbohydrates. Numerous studies have shown that carbohydrates are the main reason why a person gains weight. Carbohydrates are easily digested and converted into glucose. As has been previously illustrated, the glucose triggers insulin release, which in turn stimulates storage and weight gain. By limiting the carbohydrates, two things happen: the body has nothing to store that can add to weight and the body has to turn to fat burning in order to create the needed energy. Ketones are produced by burning fat. Thus, it is a win-win solution for the body. It gets its energy from fat while losing weight because it burns its fat storage.

Insulin is an important hormone when it comes to gaining or losing weight. This hormone signals the body to store any excess glucose. The vicious cycle goes like this:

When one eats carbohydrates, the carbohydrates are quickly converted to glucose, which immediately enters the blood. Rise in blood glucose triggers the release of insulin, in order to bring down blood sugar levels. To do so, insulin promotes glucose in the blood to be stored within the cells. Stored glucose becomes added body weight. When the blood glucose levels rapidly go down in the presence of large amounts of insulin, the body is triggered to eat more carbohydrates. This is in order to keep the blood glucose levels high and more energy available for metabolic and homeostatic processes. And the cycle starts again—more glucose, more insulin, more storage- eventually causing weight gain and obesity. By taking away carbohydrates and glucose, the body no longer has to release a lot of insulin, which means less storage, less weight gain.

Another way that makes the ketogenic diet work is from the calorie restriction. In order to induce ketosis, the body has to experience a caloric deficit. That is, the body has to be burning or requiring more energy than what it is able to take in. the best way to do this is by severely limiting carbohydrate intake.

Nutritionally speaking, fats have more calories than carbohydrates. Compare them: 1 gram of carbohydrates contains 4 calories, while 1 gram of fat contains 9 calories. However, fats are more effective in creating the caloric deficit than carbohydrates. How? Again, remember that carbohydrates are easily converted to glucose- calories that are easily used by the body. Hence, the body is programmed to rely on a steady supply of easily used glucose for energy. On the other hand, calories from fats are not easily utilized as energy. It has to undergo a longer process before it turns into an energy molecule, which in this case, is called ketones. So, while the body is still processing fat calories into energy, the body experiences a caloric deficit. It is then signaled to turn to fat stores and convert into ketone energy. The fat from the food is metabolized and stored, to replace the previously stored fat that has been recently burned. By the time that the recently consumed fat is stored, the body has already burned more for energy.

Ketogenic diets also address one of the common problems when it comes to losing weight-cravings. The body craves for sugar when it has low blood glucose levels. Again, the vicious cycle occurs. By shifting to using ketones as energy, the blood sugar levels are better regulated. That is, the body no longer puts more focus on how much glucose is in the blood because it is no longer the main energy source. With the low carbohydrate intake, the blood sugar remains at a relatively low and stable level.

Variations

Ketogenic diet has 2 main variations, in order to better address the body's needs and achieve the desired results.

TKD (targeted ketogenic diet)

This is a form of ketogenic diet that allows the dieter to eat a load of carbohydrates just before and right after a workout session. This is best for people who engage in more intense exercises. The added carbohydrates are used up immediately. This prevents depleting the glycogen stores in the muscles. This form also helps in building ore lean muscles while burning fats on a ketogenic diet.

CKD (cyclical ketogenic diet)

This form of ketogenic diet involves eating minimal carbohydrates—about 30 to 50 grams—per day, then load up on weekends. The carbohydrate loading is aimed at replenishing the glycogen stores in the liver and the muscles. This allows the person to be able to continue with intense workouts during the week.

Chapter 2 Setting Up the Diet

The main thing in ketogenic diet is to induce ketosis. This is achieved by balancing the ratios of all the macronutrients needed by the body. The ratio is determined depending on the person's age, height, weight, activity and overall health condition. Generally, the balanced ketogenic diet is consuming 60% of macronutrient requirements from fats, 35% from proteins and the small 5% is obtained from carbohydrates.

How to know that the body is indeed in ketosis

One way to check if the body is indeed in the ketotic state is checking for ketones in the urine. One popular way to do so is by using the Ketostix. Get a urine sample, dip the test strip and compare the color change to a standard color range. Ketosis is achieved when ketones are present in the urine. This means that the body is excreting excess ketones.

Another way to test is by checking the ketone levels in the blood. The test is very similar to that of taking blood glucose levels. A small blood sample is obtained from a small finger prick, placed on a test strip and inserted into a special reading device. Blood samples are best obtained during the fasted state. This would in the early morning, before taking any breakfast.

The targeted blood ketone level to induce weight loss effectively is 1.5 to 3mmol/L. Ketone levels below 0.5mmol/L is not ketosis at all. Very minimal fat burning happens at this level. Ketone levels between 0.5 and 0.15mmol/L is considered as light nutritional ketotic state, not much fat burning for weight loss. Optimum weight loss happens at 1.5 to 3.0mmol/L. Anything beyond 3mmol/L does not mean better or faster weight loss. It is actually an indication of inadequate food intake. It may also be an indication of severely low insulin levels in the body, if the person is suffering from type 1 diabetes.

Also, correct ketosis is achieved by taking the right kind of foods. Some find their ketone levels below 0.5mmol/L despite a very low carbohydrate intake, and with very minimal weight loss. This does not indicate failure of ketogenic diet. It is because of eating the wrong kinds of food.

Side Effects

For most people, the first 2 weeks of going on keto has a few discomforts. These are brought about by the body's adjustment as it shifts from being glucose-dependent to a fat-burner.

One of the best gains from going on keto diet is appetite suppression. The body learns to depend on its fat stores rather than recently consumed meals for energy. Since there is far more fat supply that provides a relatively stable supply of energy, the body feels hungry less frequently.

The drawback of the ketogenic diet is mostly seen in people that are engaged in high impact activities or in a lot of sprinting activities. These activities rely more on the quick energies provided by carbohydrates. For these people, it is recommended to go on a targeted ketogenic diet (TKD) rather than on a cyclical keto diet (CKD).

Chapter 3 Ketosis Diet Food Guide

Now, let's get to the main thing about the ketogenic diet—the food. As has been previously mentioned, carbohydrates are severely restricted and the food sources for all macronutrients should be of the right kind. Otherwise, even with limited carbohydrates, the body will not be able to achieve ketosis. Fats are to be the main energy source. Protein should be carefully balanced to provide enough building blocks for normal growth and repair of body tissues and still be within the ketotic state.

Fats

Compromising at least 60% of the daily meals, fats are the main source of calorie. It has to be from the healthy sources. Otherwise, consuming large amounts of unhealthy fats can increase the risk for health problems like cardiovascular diseases.

One thing to make sure of when taking fats is keeping a good balance between the omega-3 and omega-6 fatty acids. There should be more of the omega-3s than the omega-6s. Studies have shown that higher intake of omega-6 and less of omega-3 can actually increase the risk for chronic diseases like strokes and heart diseases. It is also linked to inflammatory conditions in the body. Good sources of omega- 3 fats are oily fishes such as wild salmon, herring, trout and tuna. Omega-6 fats are often from nuts, like macadamia nuts and walnuts. Seeds like flaxseed are rich in omega-6. It is also in abundance in nut and seed oils. Carefully use these fat sources in moderation.

Maintain a balance of saturated and monounsaturated fats. Saturated fats are often considered as the bad type of fats. In reality, it is needed by the various bodily processes. The key is to keep consumption at a minimum. Monounsaturated fats are better and healthier choices, which should comprise most of the fat requirements in the keto diet. Sources include avocado, macadamia nuts and coconut oils.

Always stay from hydrogenated or trans fats. These increase the risk for heart diseases, as they cannot be fully metabolized by the body. They clog the arteries and when oxidized, release harmful compounds like free radicals. To avoid hydrogenated fats, stay away from processed foods. These foods often have added trans fat as a preservative to extend the shelf life.

Fats can be added to meals in lots of ways. It can be used as part of the cooking process such as in frying. It can be added to sauces and dressings. It can also be as simple as adding a pat or 2 of butter over meat or steamed vegetables.

Great fat sources for ketogenic diet include the following:

- Butter

- Avocado

- Beef tallow

- Ghee

- Chicken fat (especially form the skin)

- Non hydrogenated lard

- Olive oil

- Red palm oil

- Coconut oil

- Peanut butter

- Coconut butter

Proteins

Proteins are 35% of a meal. It has to be carefully balanced because excess proteins can disrupt ketosis. The best protein sources are those from organically raised animals, grass fed and not treated with antibiotics and hormones.

Eggs are practically a mainstay in the keto diet. It is a great protein source, as well as a fat source. Choose eggs that come from organically, free-range chicken.

Other great protein sources include:

- Fish: best are those caught in the wild. Avoid "farm-raised" fish, as they tend to be fed with steroids and other harmful compounds. Also, check where the fish is caught. Stay away from those that were caught in areas with known high levels of mercury in the waters. Mercury is a toxic substance that can be obtained from eating contaminated fish and seafood. Best fishes are cod, catfish, flounder, salmon, halibut, mahi mahi, tuna, mackerel, trout and snapper.

- Shellfish: Check that these are taken from clean waters. Good protein sources, as well as of vitamins and minerals, include mussels, clams, scallops, oysters, crab, squid and lobsters.

- Pork: Best would be fresh and from organically raised pigs. Avoid processed or cured meats, because the additives are likely to contain sugars and other forms of carbohydrates. Also, processed meats may contain preservatives and other additives harmful to health. Best cuts of pork include pork chops and loin.

- Meat: Meat from grass-fed animals is better because of the higher fatty acid count. This will include beef, veal, lamb and goat.

- Poultry: choose free-range poultry such as turkey, chicken, quail, duck, pheasant

- Peanut butter is high in proteins. Eat in moderation because it is also high in carbohydrates and omega-6 fats.

Carbohydrates

This macronutrient is severely restricted in the ketogenic diet. In a day, carbohydrates consumption should be less than 50 grams. At the initiation of the ketogenic diet, carbohydrates are at 20 grams per day. This is to ensure that the body is indeed forced into ketosis. This low threshold also helps in getting a gauge of how much carbohydrates the body can go without and still function at optimum levels.

Weekend Carb Load

Some ketogenic diet variations go for a weekend carb load. That is, getting more lenient on carbohydrate consumption. Some consider this as cheat days or fun days. The weekend carb loading allows the person to "load up" by eating large quantities of carbohydrates from sources like rice, pasta, cereals, bagels, and the like, even candy.

The carbohydrates are less likely to turn to fats. Instead, it will replenish the glycogen stores in the muscles. This variation in the diet is very effective when trying to lose weight and at the same time, build lean muscle mass.

Most people find it more convenient to start weekend carbohydrate loading on Friday nights and ended before bedtime on Saturday. They can relax and enjoy the carb-loading process the entire Saturday.

If the goal is to lose weight and to build muscles, carb counting is still done even while on carb loading. To compute how much to consume, add 10 to 12 grams of carbohydrates for every kilogram of body weight. That is, a person weighing 75 kilograms is to add 750 to 900 grams carbohydrates spaced throughout the day.

The body will occasionally experience some discomfort when suddenly taking large amounts of carbohydrates after going on low-carb for some time. Dizziness and weakness will often occur, among other discomforts. To reduce these, it is advisable to take the added carbohydrates in liquid form. The best time to start is after the last workout on Friday night. At this time, the body is primed from the exercise and is ready to absorb the carbs. The body will start to adjust to the added carbohydrate load during sleep. In the morning, solid carbohydrates can be eaten without any side effects.

During weekend carb loading, keep the fat consumption at 1 gram of fat per kilogram of body weight. That is, a 75-kilo person consumes no more than 75 grams of fat during the weekend.

Vegetables

These are also important to include the diet. Vegetables may not be high in macronutrients, but are rich in phytochemicals, minerals and vitamins that can help keep the body healthy. The best vegetables for the keto diet are ones that have high nutritional contents but very low in carbs. These would be vegetables that grow above the ground. These have the least amount of starch (a form of carbohydrate) that can throw off ketosis. Great examples are dark and leafy vegetables.

Choose vegetables that are organically grown and pesticide-free. Organic and non-organic vegetables have the same nutrient content. Eating organic ones just have a lower chance of eating chemicals that may be harmful to health.

Good vegetables for keto diet include:

- Asparagus
- Broccoli
- Cauliflower
- Celery
- Lettuce

Dairy Products

Dairy products are good fat sources. Choose those that were obtained from organically raised animals and not treated with hormones and antibiotics. It is best to get the full fat variety, rather than the fat-free or low-fat ones.

Dairy products include:

- Cheeses, hard and soft: mascarpone, cheddar, cream cheese, mozzarella, and others

- Cottage cheese

- Heavy whipping cream

- Sour cream

- Buttermilk

- Milk : whole and skimmed milk

Nuts and Seeds

These are rich in proteins, omega-6 and calories. Eat in moderation. Limit consumption of nuts and seeds to a handful a day.

- Macadamia, almonds and walnuts are the best nuts to include in the ketogenic diet. Consume in moderation.

- Pistachios and cashews need to be closely checked as they are high in carbohydrates.

Nuts and seeds are better incorporated in the meals as flour. They can be substituted for refined, white flour. Examples are milled flaxseed and almond flour.

Beverages

During the first few days of starting on a keto diet, the body will lose weight due to loss of water. Carbohydrates tend to draw water towards it. When carbohydrates are stored, water is also stored. Hence, aside from the weight of stored carbohydrates, the water retained also contributes to weight gain. In the absence of carbohydrates, the body starts to release retained water.

This is the diuretic effect of the ketogenic diet. It also puts a person at risk for dehydration. That is why it is important to keep hydrated. But one has to be careful of the beverages. Some may contain carbohydrates that disrupt ketosis.

The best way to keep hydrated is taking water. In a day, take at least 8 glasses of water or 1.5 to 2 liters. Drink all throughout the day and then some until evening.

Coffee and tea can also be consumed while on keto diet. Just make sure to include any added cream or sugars (artificial or natural sweeteners) to the carb and fat count.

Chapter 4 Ketogenic Recipes

Here are ketogenic recipes to get you started.

For breakfast

Ketogenic Bacon and Eggs

Ingredients:

- 8 slices of bacon, the meaty type
- 1 tablespoon organic butter
- ½ cup cauliflower or broccoli flowerets, chopped
- 1 medium-sized carrot, peeled into thin strips
- ½ large white onion, chopped
- ½ cup celery, chopped finely
- ½ cup Colby jack cheese, shredded
- 4 large eggs, preferably organic

Procedure:

1. Slice the bacon into small strips. Slice across the direction of the grain.

2. Place a large skillet over medium heat. Melt the butter. Add the bacon strips and all the vegetables.

3. Sauté the vegetables and bacon, stirring frequently. Cook until the edges of the bacon start to crisp and the vegetables caramelize. This will take about 20 minutes.

4. Divide the bacon-vegetable mix into four. Make a well in the middle of each of the portions. Take one of the eggs and break it in the middle of the well.

5. Cook the eggs until desired.

6. When the eggs are almost done, sprinkle cheese on top. Cook for a few more minutes until the cheese melts.

Serve hot.

Baked Breakfast Bacon and Eggs

Ingredients:

- 4 large eggs
- 8 slices bacon, cooked and crumbled
- 2 tablespoons butter
- 1 cup heavy cream, heat until lukewarm
- 1 cup cheddar cheese, grated
- salt and pepper to taste

Procedure:

1. Turn the oven and preheat to 350°F.

2. Get 4 6-oz ramekins and butter them. (approximately half a teaspoon per ramekin)

3. Break an egg in each ramekin.

4. On top of the egg, place ¼ cup cheese and ¼ cup of the heated cream. Season with salt and pepper.

5. Place the ramekins in a shallow baking pan. Add enough water to the pan until the water reaches half up the side of the ramekins.

6. Place the pan into the oven and bake for 15 minutes or until the cheese melts and the egg whites are no longer translucent.

7. Remove from the oven and top with crumbled bacon before serving.

Low Carb Breakfast Fruit Muffins

Ingredients (makes 15 muffins):

- 2 cups almond flour or other nut/seed flour
- ½ teaspoon baking soda
- 5 packets artificial sweetener (Splenda or Stevia)
- 1 cup heavy cream
- 1/8 cup butter, melted
- 2 large eggs
- ½ teaspoon lemon flavoring or extract
- ¼ teaspoon sea or rock salt
- ½ teaspoon dried lemon zest
- 4 ounces of fresh blueberries

Procedure:

1. Preheat the oven to 350°F degrees.
2. Prepare a muffin tray. Place cupcake papers over the muffin holes.
3. Mix the flour and cream.
4. And the eggs, one at a time. Mix well after each addition.
5. Add butter, sweetener of choice and baking soda.
6. Add the flavorings (salt, lemon zest and extract).
7. Add the blueberries. Mix well until the blueberries are evenly distributed in the muffin mixture.

8. Spoon the mixture into the muffin tray. Fill it ½ full.

9. Bake in the oven for 20 minutes or until the muffin turns a golden color.

10. Remove from the oven and cool on a separate tray.

11. Serve warm with a pat of butter.

*Nutritional content (per muffin): 184 calories

5 grams of protein, 17 grams of fat, 6 grams of carbohydrates, 2 gram of fiber (net carb 4 grams)

Savory Keto Cheese Muffins

Ingredients (makes 12 muffins):

- 2 cups almond flour☐☐
- ¼ teaspoon salt
- ½ teaspoon baking soda
- 1 cup sour cream
- 2 large eggs
- 1/8 cup organic butter, melted
- ½ teaspoon dried thyme
- ½ cup muenster, shredded
- 1 cup shredded cheddar or Colby jack

Procedure:

1. Preheat the oven to 400°F.
2. Prepare the muffin tray by placing cupcake liners.
3. In a bowl, combine almond flour and the rest of the dry ingredients. Give the mixture a quick whisk.
4. Get another bowl. Lightly beat the eggs. Add the sour cream and melted butter.
5. Gradually add the liquid mixture into the dry mixture. Mix thoroughly. If the mix seems too dry, add 1 tablespoon of heavy cream or water at a time until the desired consistency is achieved.
6. Add the cheese and mix until evenly distributed.

7. Spoon the mixture into the muffin tray, filling only ¾ full.

8. Bake in the oven at 400°F for about 5 minutes.

9. Reduce the temperature to 350°F. Bake for 20 minutes more until the muffin turns golden brown.

10. Remove from the oven and let cool. Serve with a pat of butter.

*Nutrition content per muffin: 166 calories

6 grams of protein, 15 grams of fat, 5 grams of carbohydrates with 3 grams of fiber (net carb 2 grams for each muffin)

Strawberry Almond Smoothie

Ingredients (makes 2 servings):

- 16 ounces almond milk, unsweetened
- 4 ounces heavy cream
- 1 packet artificial sweetener (Stevia or Splenda)
- 1 scoop whey powder
- 1/4 cup frozen strawberries, unsweetened

Procedure:

1. Combine all ingredients in a blender.
2. Blend until smooth and well mixed.
3. Add a little water if the mixture is too thick.

*Nutrition content (per serving): 304 calories

15 grams of protein, 25 grams of fat, 7 grams carbohydrates, 1 gram fiber (net carb 6 grams)

For lunch/dinner

Baked Chicken with Herbed Cream Sauce

Ingredients (makes 4 servings):

- 5 tablespoons butter, divided
- 3 large garlic cloves
- 1 teaspoon dried tarragon
- 2 small white onions, sliced thinly
- ½ cup chicken broth
- ½ cup heavy cream
- ½ cup dry white wine
- 8 oz cream cheese
- 1 ½ teaspoon herbes de Provence
- 4 raw chicken breasts
- 1 teaspoon chicken seasoning (check for carbs on label)
- Salt to taste

Procedure:

1. Place a skillet over medium heat. Melt 2 tablespoons of butter. Sauté tarragon, onions and garlic until soft. Remove from the skillet. Set aside.

2. Add 2 more tablespoon of butter to the same skillet. Add the wine and cream cheese. Mix until the cheese melts and the mixture becomes uniform in consistency.

3. Add the cream and other spices.

4. Preheat the oven to 350°F.

5. Grease a glass baking dish (measuring 9 inches by 13 inches) with the remaining 1 tablespoon of butter.

6. Pour the chicken broth into the baking dish.

7. Arrange the chicken breast in a single layer in the baking dish.

8. Add the sautéed onions, tarragon and garlic over the chicken.

9. Pour the cream sauce evenly over the chicken and onions.

10. Bake in the oven for 45 minutes to 1 hour.

11. Remove from the oven.

12. Serve warm with fresh garden salad.

*Nutrition content (per serving): 478 calories

11 grams protein, 46 grams fat, 5 grams carbohydrates, 1 gram fiber (net carb 4 grams)

Baked Herbed Salmon

Ingredients:

- 2 pounds salmon fillets
- ½ cup tamari soy sauce
- 4 ounces sesame oil
- 1 teaspoon minced garlic
- ½ teaspoon basil
- ½ teaspoon ground ginger
- 1 teaspoon oregano leaves
- ½ teaspoon rosemary
- ¼ teaspoon thyme
- ¼ teaspoon tarragon
- 4 ounces butter
- ½ cup green onions, chopped
- ½ cup fresh mushrooms, chopped

Procedure:

1. Mix sesame oil, tamari sauce and all the herbs and spices to make the marinade.

2. Put the salmon fillets in a freezer bag or resealable plastic bag. Pour the marinade in. Lightly massage the fish to let the marinade sink in.

3. Marinade the salmon with the skin side up inside the refrigerator for 1 to 4 hours.

4. Preheat the oven to 350°F. Get a large, shallow baking pan and line it with foil.

5. Get the fish and arrange it in a single layer on the baking dish. Pour the marinade over the fish.

6. Bake in the oven for 10 to 15 minutes.

7. In a large skillet, melt the butter.

8. Add the onions and mushrooms. Mix until everything is coated with butter.

9. Remove the salmon from the oven and pour the buttered onion and mushroom on top of the fish. Makes sure that each fillet is covered.

10. Return to the oven and bake for another 10 minutes.

11. Serve immediately once done.

*Nutrition content (per 8-ounce serving): 353 calories

32 grams protein, 23 grams fat, 2 grams carbohydrates, 1 gram of fiber (net carb 1 gram)

Baked Lemon Salmon

Ingredients:

- 2 pieces 6-ounce salmon fillets
- 6 tablespoons light olive oil
- 1 tablespoon lemon juice
- 2 cloves garlic, minced
- 1 tablespoon fresh parsley, chopped
- 1 teaspoon dried basil
- 1 teaspoon salt
- 1 teaspoon ground black pepper

Procedure:

1. Prepare the marinade in a medium glass bowl. Mix the olive oil, basil, garlic, lemon juice, pepper, parsley and salt.

2. Place the salmon fillets in a medium-sized glass baking dish.

3. Pour the marinade over the fish.

4. Marinade for an hour inside the refrigerator. Turn occasionally, about once every 30 minutes.

5. Preheat the oven to 375°F.

6. Arrange the salmon filets on a piece of aluminum foil. Pour marinade over the fish and seal the foil.

7. Place the wrapped salmon in a glass baking dish. Bake in the oven for 35 to 45 minutes or until the fish easily flakes when pierced with a fork.

8. Remove from the oven and serve immediately.

*Nutrition content (for each 6-ounce serving): 436 calories

37 grams protein, 30 grams fat, 2 grams carbohydrates, 1 gram fiber (net carb 1 gram)

Baked Cauliflower with Cheddar

Ingredients (makes 4 servings):

- 1 medium-sized cauliflower head

- 3 tablespoon crème fraiche

- 2 large eggs

- 50 grams cheddar cheese, grated

- 1.5 liters water

- 1 tablespoon olive oil

- Mixture of cumin seeds, garlic and hot chili, according to desired amount

- Salt and pepper to taste

Procedure:

1. Preheat the oven to 390°F.

2. Boil the 1.5 liters of water.

3. Add the spices.

4. Separate the cauliflower flowerets. Add them to the boiling water.

5. Simmer the cauliflower for 3 minutes then drain. Place in ice bath to retain crispness and vibrant color.

6. Prepare the baking dish. Lightly grease with butter or oil.

7. Arrange the cauliflower in the bottom of the baking dish. Set aside.

8. In a separate bowl, whisk the eggs. Add the olive oil and crème fraiche.

9. Pour the cream mixture evenly over the cauliflower.

10. Top with grated cheese.

11. Bake in the oven for 15 to 20 minutes.

12. Grill for another 1 to 2 minutes for a thicker and golden crust.

13. Remove from the oven and serve hot or chilled.

*Nutrition content (per serving): 204 kcal

16 grams fat, 9.5 grams protein, 8.5 grams carbohydrates, 3.5 grams fiber (net carb 5 grams)

For Dessert/Snack

Ketogenic Pudding

Ingredients (makes 3 servings):

- 4 ounces heavy whipping cream

- 8 ounces cream cheese, softened

- 1 tablespoon sugar free syrup, flavor depending on preference

- 4-6 drops liquid Stevia or EZ-Sweet, to taste

Procedure:

1. Combine all ingredients.

2. Mix until smooth in consistency.

3. Divide the mixture in 3 serving bowls.

4. Chill in the refrigerator until the pudding sets.

5. Serve.

*Nutrition content (per 1-ounce serving): 401 calories

7 grams protein, 41 grams fat, 3 grams carbohydrates

Conclusion

Thank you again for purchasing this book!

I hope this book was able to help you to understand what the ketogenic diet is all about. It is not just a fad diet or a crash diet. It is a diet that promotes better health through better eating habits.

The next step is to remove all the unhealthy foods from your home. Start buying healthier food items and start living keto starting today. Tell everyone just how wonderful this diet is. Best of all, be the living proof that this diet does work.

Finally, if you enjoyed this book, please take the time to share your thoughts and post a positive review on Amazon. It'd be greatly appreciated!

In addition, please remember to check out our Facebook page in order to find other resources and upcoming promotions:

https://www.facebook.com/joypublishing

With sincere thanks,

Emma Rose

Preview Of "Paleo Free Diet Guide for Beginners: Over 50 Paleo Free Diet Recipes for Fast Weight Loss and Optimal Health"

Introduction

I want to thank you and congratulate you for purchasing the book, *"Paleo Free Diet Guide for Beginners: Over 50 Paleo Free Diet Recipes for Optimal Health and Fast Weight Loss"*.

This book contains everything you might need to know when it comes to getting started with the Paleo diet. It is provided in an easily digestible format that allows you to better absorb the information. There are no complicated explanations about how it works! You'll be given what you need straight up so you won't have to waste time trying to understand exactly what the diet is. Whether it's for your overall good health or to lose a few pounds, Paleo can certainly help you with it. To help you get started, we'll do the same and start you off with 50 of the best Paleo recipes that you can slowly but surely shift your everyday menu to.

It's never easy changing a diet. I often fall into self pity when I can no longer have the foods I enjoy. Either I feel sorry for myself or I get rebellious and binge and anything and everything. I always knew the value of eating healthy. I could just never bring myself to do it. It wasn't until I had a miscarriage that I got serious about my health. I have made drastic changes that others just don't understand. But the pay off is the weight I've lost and the better health I'm experiencing.

My hope for you is not to be on another "diet." This isn't a restriction diet like Atkins. The goal is to have a lifestyle change. Lifestyle changes are more sustainable and maintain weight loss long term compared to restriction diets. The change is hard to start but worth it when you commit. The trick is to get the momentum to start.

Thanks again for purchasing this book. I hope you enjoy reading it and eating the recipes from it!

With gratitude,

Emma Rose

Chapter 1 – What Is the Paleo Diet?

The Paleo Diet is known by many names such as the cavemen diet, stone age diet and hunter-gatherer diet, to name a few. The concept behind this diet follows that of the Paleolithic era before the development of agriculture. Essentially, you consume the same foods that the cavemen used to eat. The focus is on eating food closest to its natural, unprocessed state. The cavemen would gather their food from any source available whether it was wild animals, berries, vegetables, or fruits. As a result, they were strong, fit, and healthy for thousands of years.

This type of diet is still very young, less than fifty years only, but more in depth researches and studies are being conducted to increase the information and knowledge on this diet. The results of previous studies conducted on the Paleo diet reveal the improvement of health to the people involved. This is attributed to the fact that no processed foods and additives are included. The Paleo Diet is a diet that works with our genetics – before machinery and processing got involved. Foods that were not available during the Paleolithic time such as dairy products, salt, sugar and grains are not included in the preparation of the Paleo diet.

The modern diet predominately consumed in the Western world is full of refined foods, trans fats, salt and sugar. These ingredients are known to indirectly cause diseases such as hypertension, diabetes, strokes, obesity and other heart problems. The list goes on even further with the increase diagnosis of cancer, Parkinson's, Alzheimer's, depression and infertility. "What an extraordinary achievement for a civilization: to have developed the one diet that reliably makes its people sick!" (Michael Pollen, Food Rules: An Eater's Manual, Penguin Books 2009).

Foods included in the Paleo Diet

- Fruit

- Vegetables

- Lean Meat

- Seafood

- Nuts/Seeds

- Healthy Fats (eg. coconut, avocado, nuts and seeds, olive oil, grass fed butter)

Foods NOT included in the Paleo Diet

- Dairy

- Grain

- Processed Food

Why not grain?

You may be surprised to see that grains are not included in the Paleo Diet. We are accustomed to grains being a part of a balanced diet. However, our bodies are not designed to deal with the nutritional components of grains such as gluten, lectin, and phytates.

Gluten is a protein substance found in wheat, barley and rye. Many people are discovering that their bodies are gluten sensitive and are eliminating gluten from their diet. The most extreme case of gluten sensitivity is Celiac Disease. Individuals with this disease can pick up the minutest trace of gluten and react immediately.

Lectin binds to insulin receptors and can also cause leptin resistance.

Phytates cause minerals to become unavailable during digestion.

Check out the rest of "Paleo Free Diet Guide for Beginners: Over 50 Paleo Diet Recipes for Fast Weight Loss and Optimal Health" on Amazon

Or go to: http://amzn.to/1jIJUFX

Detox Diet Guide

Lose Weight Quickly, Achieve Optimal Health and Feel Energized Through the 10 Day Detox

Emma Rose

Table of Contents

Introduction

I want to thank you and congratulate you for purchasing the book, *"Detox Diet Guide: Lose Weight Quickly, Achieve Optimal Health and Feel Energized Through the 10 Day Detox"*.

This book contains proven steps and strategies on how to not just simply flush out toxic substances from our bodies, but to also enhance the way our bodies naturally flush out those toxins.

It also contains other important information such as the most common toxins that are found in the environment that we unknowingly consume, the many ways our bodies naturally detoxify themselves, the things one must and must not do within the ten days of the detox diet, detoxification recipes that can be easily prepared, and some important reminders that must be taken before, during, and after the detox diet.

Thanks again for purchasing this book. I hope you enjoy it! Please take some time to stop by and LIKE our Facebook page:

https://www.facebook.com/joypublishing

With gratitude,

Emma Rose

Chapter 1: Toxins and the Body

As the human body does its usual processes, some things need to be expelled. These are usually waste products made as a result of filtering out substances not needed by the body. There is a reason for the so-called "calls of nature" – which are peeing and releasing excrement.

But sometimes, those unwanted substances can build up in the organs and the bodily systems that comprise them. If there are too much of those substances, they will cause all sorts of harm to the overall bodily functions that can lead to various ailments.

The Top 10 List of Most Common Toxins

Human civilization evolves as a result of the desire of the people to live more comfortably and conveniently. But in the process of that evolution, it has unknowingly unleashed a cavalcade of impurities that do not just pollute the environment, but also the human body. Despite the many efforts by several government agencies and private individuals to thwart the sources of those impurities, there are traces of those impurities that still linger around. Those traces remain in the air, in the soil, in several bodies of water – and eventually, in the foods that humanity consumes.

According to Dr. Joseph Mercola, a well-known personality in the US wellness movement and owner and founder of Mercola.com (one of the most-trusted health websites), the ten most common toxic substances that are still prevalent in the environment to this day are the following:

1. Polychlorinated biphenyls, or PCBs, were commonly dumped by factories into nearby bodies of water. Due to their toxicity, PCBs were banned decades ago. However, traces of PCBs can still be found in those bodies of water since the toxic substances do not break down easily even after all those years. Fish that swim in those bodies of water still consume PCBs

unknowingly. As people still eat those fish, they will also ingest PCBs that will contribute to ailments such as cancer and brain defects in newborn babies.

2. Pesticides, while they do kill pests as their name says, are the major contributors of cancer. As farms still use synthetic pesticides such as weed killers, fungi killers, and insect killers; residues of those pesticides still remain in as much as 50 to 90 percent of US farm produce. Furthermore, there are bug sprays used to kill cockroaches and other unwanted insects in homes. Those bug sprays also contain the same carcinogenic substances as farm-focused pesticides. Besides cancer, pesticides also cause Parkinson's disease, miscarriage, nerve damage, birth defects, and getting in the way of nutrient absorption.

3. Fungal toxins not just come in the form of poisonous mushrooms. The most common of those fungal toxins is mould. Mould thrives in moist places such as bathrooms and kitchens; and can even sustain in vulnerable foods such as peanuts, wheat, and corn. One in three people are allergic to this fungal toxin. If left unchecked, mould causes cancer, heart disease, asthma, multiple sclerosis, and diabetes.

4. Phthalates are commonly found in plastic products and are responsible for softening them, making them easier to mold. They can seep into foodstuffs and drinks that are placed inside plastic food containers and plastic bottles. The result of ingesting too much phthalates is hormonal imbalance, since the substances resemble naturally-produced hormones. In children, phthalates can stunt their growth.

5. Volatile organic compounds, or VOCs, are commonly found in several household products such as air fresheners, cleaning fluids, mothballs, and varnishes. VOCs aid in air pollution and cause several sicknesses such as cancer, irritation of eyes and lungs, headaches, dizziness, and impaired memory.

6. Dioxins are some of the pollutants that are produced when something is burned, especially in massive quantities. As they

are released into the air, humans not just breathe in the dioxins. Livestock can also inhale those toxins and settle in their fats even after they are brought to the slaughterhouse to be made into meat. Dioxins cause cancer, stunted growth, reproductive system impairments, skin disorders such as acne, and slight damage to the liver.

7. Asbestos was a popular insulation material, but it was banned in the seventies due to its carcinogenic effects. Traces of asbestos can still be found in old homes that did not have their insulations replaced. Besides cancer, asbestos causes scarring on the lung tissue.

8. Toxic heavy metals such as lead, arsenic, and mercury can still be found in various objects such as cheaply-made toys, preserved wood, antiperspirants, and building materials. Once those metals are inhaled or ingested, they can cause cancer, brain and nerve disorders such as Alzheimer's disease, nausea, lesser amounts of red and white blood cells, and abnormal heartbeats.

9. Chloroform is a common chemical that is used to make other chemicals. It is prevalent in the air, in water, and in food. It can cause cancer, infertility, birth defects, headaches, dizziness, and damage to the liver and kidneys.

10. Chlorine is commonly found in water as it is used to purify it. Whether from the typical drinking water or from a swimming pool, too much of chlorine will cause all sorts of respiratory problems such as sore throat, accumulation of fluid in the lungs, and asthma.

Based on this list, many of those toxins in the environment are brought about by humanity's modern lifestyles. Before they do undue harm to the body, especially the dreaded cancer, they must be flushed out promptly.

Other Sources of Toxins

Besides the ten most common toxic substances, there are also other toxins that can be found in almost everything in the modern world. It is inevitable that one must intake those toxins unknowingly, one way or the other.

The two most popular vices, which are smoking and drinking, are the other major reasons for the body's toxicity. Both alcohol and nicotine have been proven many times by the scientific community to be not just toxic, but also addicting. Those two substances also alter the brain's functions. Other toxic substances include caffeine, empty sugars, and saturated fats. The latter two are especially notorious for being fat fodder since they cannot be processed into needed energy.

Many cosmetics today also contain toxic substances such as VOCs that can be absorbed into the skin. Some cosmetics producers have already taken steps in ridding their beauty products of those toxins.

Taking too many medications all at once can also cause the body to be laced with toxins, since they are not properly eliminated from the body. If the body feels too taxed from a cornucopia of meds, a consultation with the doctor will help.

There are also naturally-occurring toxins that are used by certain plants and animals as defense mechanisms against invaders. Snakes and jellyfish have highly deadly toxins and should not be consumed as food. A Japanese dish called *fugu* uses a type of blowfish that releases toxins which will certainly kill someone who eats an improperly-prepared version of the dish.

Processed foods, especially canned goods, are also a major source of toxins. While those foods contain preservatives that prolong their shelf lives, they unknowingly unleash a world of hurt on one who voraciously eats these. Needless to say, one must balance those foods out with naturally-grown foods.

Chapter 2: Why Must We Detoxify?

Detoxification is not just the simple flushing out of unwanted substances when the body cannot handle expelling them on its own. It is also the purging of impure thoughts in the mind that cause all sorts of decisions to inhale and ingest several toxins, whether knowingly or unknowingly, into the body. To ensure that an individual is rightfully clean in both body and mind, all sorts of unwanted things must be eliminated, especially in the detox diet.

The Body Does It Own Job...

The excretory system does its job of purging waste substances from the body via its two major processes: urination and release of excrement. Urination is obviously handled by the urinary system, while the release of excrement is handled by the lower parts of the digestive system.

The urinary system's main actor is the kidneys. The kidneys filter unwanted stuff such as ammonia, urea, uric acid, and excess salt and water from the blood as well as other bodily fluids. Those unwanted stuff then get to the bladder, which acts as a temporary storage. If the bladder gets full, the stuff gets expelled out of the urethra in the form of urine. Ammonia is a byproduct of the breakdown and usage of protein for the body's energy, while urea and uric acid are less toxic substances that result from the breakdown of ammonia.

The lower parts of the digestive system consist of the liver, the intestines, and the colon. The liver does its job of breaking down foreign substances so that the kidneys can have an easier job filtering them out as urine. The intestines and the colon facilitate the expelling of solid waste substances in the form of feces. The colon, in particular, absorbs trace minerals such as potassium and sends them to the bloodstream before they are included as feces that will be expelled by pooping.

Another natural detoxifier found in the human body is the lymphatic system. The lymphatic system contains lymph nodes that are scattered throughout the body but are interconnected. Those nodes provide the body with immunity, complementing the immune system, by filtering out unwelcome invaders such as bacteria, viruses, old red blood cells, and other toxic substances.

Other parts of the excretory system consist of the lungs and skin. The lungs expel excess water and carbon dioxide when someone breathes out. The skin kicks out excess water, salt, uric acid, and excess trace minerals in the form of sweat.

...But It Is Not Enough in the Modern Age

However, as demonstrated in the previous chapter, there are far too many substances that are deemed toxic in the wrong amounts. With humanity's modern lifestyles, the body does not know what to make of the increasing number of unwelcome invaders in its insides. These usually never get flushed out as urine and feces, but instead accumulate in the body fat.

As the invaders multiply and never get flushed out, they get in the way of the body's usual processes and will cause several problems such as depleted energy levels, unnatural weight gain, and various diseases that target the major body systems.

Another thing that is not helping the body in its natural detoxification process is the busy and hectic schedules people normally have. Because those people have no time to perform even mundane healthy tasks such as drinking adequate water, the body never gets its supply of natural detox assistants. Couple the lack of those assistants with stress and it will be a recipe for disaster.

Therefore, it is important that in this world of toxicity, people must amplify their bodily defenses against all sorts of foreign toxic substances by enhancing the many components of the excretory system such as the kidneys, the liver, the intestines, and the colon. With the contaminants out of the way, the body's natural healing processes also get their groove back. As the major organ systems work hand-in-hand, the benefits that are felt in one particular system will spread towards the other systems.

In short, steeling the body and its functions, especially the excretory functions, is one of the first lines of defense against toxin-induced sicknesses. There will be a marked loss in weight, since the excessive fats as well as the toxins they contain are properly expelled. There will also be renewed liveliness since the bodily functions that have something to do with the intake and processing of energy sources are no longer clogged by invasive toxins.

Why the Mind Is Also Important in Detoxification

The decisions a person makes, no matter how small they are, can contribute to huge consequences. For example, if one decides to commute to a bar, he or she gets all sorts of toxins in the process – airborne impurities from urban roads, food additives from the snacks he or she eats while commuting, nicotine and other chemicals from tobacco smoke generated by smokers inside and outside the bar, and alcohol from the hard drinks he or she consumes while in the bar.

Therefore, it is important that a person must think thoroughly and deeply before settling on a decision that will make him or her take in all those unwanted toxins along the way. Yes, this may turn him or her into a control freak, but there are also decisions that will endow him or her with long-term benefits. Remember, detoxification starts in the mind. The decisions that lead to the unknowing intake of toxins must be sorted out and eliminated from the usual routines first.

Chapter 3: The Crucial Ten Days

There are several forms of detoxification, and they more often than not involve ingesting special liquids and solids, cleansing the colon, foot baths and foot pads, spas and saunas, and fasting. But they also cost money, are always focused on the short-term effects, and may not deliver the detoxification results one desires. The best form of the detox diet must involve getting rid of major sources of toxins, ingesting more of the substances that will greatly assist the body's natural detoxification processes, never integrating any form of starvation or elimination of a major food group from the diet, and clearing the mind of impure thoughts that lead to impure actions. This way, the diet will grant long-term effects of well-being. As a beneficial consequence, this diet will cost little to no money, except for the money to be spent on detoxifying foods and drinks.

The ten days this detox diet contains are important to ensure natural weight loss and general well-being. And even after the diet period ends, some good habits contained in this diet, particularly the continued eating of healthy foods, must still be kept. This is to ensure that the person undergoing this diet will transition into a healthy lifestyle.

Preparing for the Diet

One important thing to do when undergoing this diet, or any other diet for that matter, is to not rush in immediately. A crash diet will have nasty consequences such as abrupt changing of body patterns that lead to all sorts of ailments as well as retention of the weight one lost during the diet routine. Therefore, one must start slow and transition into the diet carefully.

Not rushing in also applies to the chewing of food. The body needs some time to digest the food. Never treat the ten days of the diet like some kind of work deadline.

The usual vice-based sources of toxins, which are tobacco and alcohol, must be eliminated first. While dealing with the withdrawal effects of both of those substances may be difficult, timely help from a doctor who has a specialization in several types of addictions and substance abuse will lessen the difficulty.

In the three days before the actual start of the diet, rid the pantry and fridge of tempting foodstuffs that are loaded with empty calories. These include sweets and most forms of processed foods and fast food. At the same time, steadily increase the intake of fruits and vegetables – *especially organic ones*. As much as possible, turn the veggies into freshly-prepared salads and/or lightly steam them. As for the fruits, eat them raw and/or turn them into natural juices.

Since pesticide residue in fruits and vegetables is inevitable, the use of fruit and vegetable washes must be prioritized.

The intake of caffeine must be slowly and surely reduced to prevent withdrawal symptoms such as headaches. Switching to decaf coffee and low-caffeine teas such as green tea will help, as is the trick of diluting regular coffee and tea in huge amounts of water.

And speaking of water, the time-tested advice of eight to ten glasses of water a day will especially help the detox diet become successful. Drink it throughout the ten days of the diet.

Aromatherapy using essential oils is helpful, as this therapy helps to calm the mind in order for it to prepare for the rigors of the critical ten days.

Finally, before embarking on the detox diet itself, please consult a registered dietician who can recommend the detoxifying foods to be eaten based on your genetic makeup. Furthermore, *do not stop* taking prescribed medicine, as discontinuing medications can have devastating effects on the body. Diets are not meant to be one-man shows, especially if the individual still has to learn much about the intricacies of diet programs like this.

Eat and Drink Them

With the transition phase over, it is time to actually start the detox diet. Here is a comprehensive list of foods and drinks that must be ingested during the ten crucial days of the diet.

1. Organic fruits and vegetables are the main focus of the detox diet. It does not matter what the size or type of fruit or vegetable one will be consuming – as long as it is free of pesticides and synthetic fertilizers and is grown using age-old farming techniques, it certainly counts. Eat a good variety of fruits and vegetables to round out all the necessary nutrients.

2. Brown rice is much healthier compared to the typical white rice. As white rice is a result of the milling process, brown rice retains some nutrients that are usually lost during milling. This type of rice is also a rich source of fiber, which will aid in flushing the toxins out via the intestines and the colon.

3. Herbs are permissible, since they are also plants. Use them to flavor the dishes as well as utilize them for aromatherapy. Herbal teas are also a-OK, since they do not contain caffeine at all. As with fruits and vegetables, herbs must not have traces of anything toxic.

4. Whole-grain products, much like brown rice, do not undergo the nutrient-losing milling process. They are also rich sources of fiber. Whole-grain products include whole wheat bread, bran, and rolled oats.

5. Seaweeds such as kelp and *nori* wrappers used for sushi are also plant-based. They can also be consumed the same way as typical veggies do.

6. Beans such as green peas, chick peas, lentils, kidney beans, and black beans are permitted.

7. One can go nuts with nuts and seeds. Allowable things include almonds, cashews, walnuts, watermelon seeds, pumpkin

13

seeds, sunflower seeds, and sesame seeds. As a general rule, pick only raw, unsalted nuts and seeds.

8. Coconuts, while they are not actually nuts, are also allowed. There are several coconut-based consumables such as coconut water and coconut oil. One can also eat fresh coconut meat straight from the source.

9. Plant-based oils are encouraged. Olive oil, especially the extra virgin kind, is highly recommended.

10. Round out the protein-based nutrition with plant-based protein sources such as soy. Soy milk and tofu are easily-acquired sources of plant-based protein.

11. All sorts of edible mushrooms are permitted. Portobello and shiitake mushrooms can act as good substitutes for meat.

12. Natural sweeteners such as raw honey and natural maple syrup are permitted.

13. Besides herbs, other natural condiments that are tolerable include apple cider vinegar, sea salt, and mustard.

14. If there is still a desire to eat meat and get adequate protein, go with lean meats such as fish and organic chicken. Eggs are also on the list, as long as they are organic.

Never Eat and Drink Them

Meanwhile, these are the foods and drinks to avoid during the detox diet phase.

1. In general, non-lean types of red meat are off-limits. Canned meat is especially forbidden.

2. All forms of processed foods containing all sorts of additives and preservatives are out of the question. On a related note, artificial sweeteners and processed condiments are also out.

3. Typical white sugar and brown sugar are verboten, as well as high-fructose syrups.

4. Corn must be avoided as it is acid-forming. The acid in question is uric acid. Furthermore, the corn kernels that are indigestible will make bathroom breaks more excruciating.

5. While nuts are OK, peanuts and peanut butter are usually excluded.

6. Milk is normally not allowed, but half a cup of yogurt containing good bacteria per day is an exception to that.

7. Caffeine is another typical forbidden substance.

8. Shortening and margarine are inadmissible.

9. While fish is OK, other seafoods are not.

Other Cleansing Procedures

There are many variations of the detox diet, but the one being presented in this book will not involve complicated doohickeys and specialized food and drinks to amplify the detoxification effect. Here are some things one can also do during the ten days of the diet.

With all the conveniences of Internet-based connectivity, sometimes too much is too much. Dedicate one of the ten days, or even all ten days, to a temporary break from technology. Put away the smartphone or tablet, avoid touching the computer, and never be tempted to go online just about anywhere. Take the time off from technology to visit someplace serene, like a retreat house. This technology break will clear the mind of all sorts of burdening thoughts that may poison one's thinking the same way that bodily toxins do.

Take some time off to scrape the tongue. Tongue scraping is a practice in ayurvedic medicine, or ancient Hindu medicine, where all the impurities built up on the tongue are removed. Tongue scrapers can be bought for cheap at drug store.

Try to write all the stored thoughts and feelings, even negative ones, into a diary or notebook. Releasing all the stored strong emotions to a diary or notebook has a cathartic effect, since keeping those emotions locked away will eventually take the toll on one's health.

Another mind-cleansing procedure one can do during the ten days is meditation. Meditation also helps clear the mind of toxic thoughts that lead to stress, which then slows down the liver's detoxification process. Yoga is especially helpful as a meditation tool. You may also augment your meditation by doing deep breathing exercises or visualizing relaxing images such as watching the sunset at the beach.

Get enough dosages of vitamin C. While the vitamin is better known for boosting immunity, it also helps the body with the production of glutathione. Glutathione may be better known as a skin rejuvenating agent, but it also exists in the liver as a detoxification aid. Citrus fruits are the best-known sources of vitamin C.

Enhance blood circulation, since poor blood circulation will hamper the flushing out of impurities from the blood. Exercise is a guaranteed way to get that blood pumping.

Keep in mind that not all bacteria are bad. Good bacteria mostly reside in the intestines, aiding in digestion and preventing bad bacteria from releasing toxins that can be deployed in the bloodstream. Help the good bacteria by taking probiotic drinks.

Chapter 4: Detoxification Recipes

Breakfast Recipes

Gut-Busting Oatmeal Bowl

Ingredients:

- 1-2 cups oatmeal

- 1-2 cups water or nut milk

- A mixture of fresh berries and fresh fruits, all sliced

Procedure:

1. Prepare the oatmeal as indicated in the packaging.

2. While hot, pour the berries and fruits onto the prepared oatmeal, and mix.

Berry Blast Smoothie

Ingredients:

- 1-2 cups mixed fresh berries
- 1-2 cups protein powder
- 1-2 cups ice cubes

Procedure:

1. Throw all the ingredients into a blender, and hit puree.

2. Serve the smoothie in a tall glass.

Lunch Recipes

Veggie Cavalcade Salad with Tofu

Ingredients:

- 6-8 pieces of any whole vegetable (for greens, an amount of at least five leaves equals one whole piece)

- 1-2 pieces tofu, diced

- 4-5 teaspoons extra virgin olive oil

- 2 teaspoons fresh lemon juice

- 1 teaspoon freshly-chopped herbs of choice

Procedure:

1. Fry the tofu in 2-3 teaspoons olive oil until slightly browned. Set aside.

2. Slice and/or dice the vegetables into reasonably-sized pieces. Leave the greens untouched.

3. Pour all the vegetables and the tofu into a bowl. Mix completely.

4. Combine 2 teaspoons olive oil, the lemon juice, and the herbs to make the dressing.

5. Pour the dressing all over the salad. Mix completely.

Special Omelet Rice

Ingredients:

- 3-5 organic eggs
- Fresh or dried herbs (any variety), to taste
- 2-3 teaspoons extra virgin olive oil
- 1-2 cups cooked brown rice

Procedure:

1. Beat the eggs into a scramble while adding the herbs.

2. Pour the olive oil into a heated pan. Wait until the oil is hot.

3. Pour the egg and herb mixture until the omelet is formed. Turn over to ensure proper cooking.

4. Once the omelet is out of the pan, place the brown rice inside it. Make sure the omelet wraps around the rice.

5. Serve hot with mustard.

Dinner Recipes

The Steamed Medley

Ingredients:

- 1 slice salmon

- 5-10 pieces broccoli and asparagus (can be of any combination)

- 1/4 cup fresh lemon juice

- Fresh or dried herbs (any variety), to taste

Procedure:

1. In a steamer or a rice cooker with a steaming basket, arrange the salmon slice and the broccoli and asparagus pieces so that the steam will be evenly distributed.

2. Sprinkle the salmon and the vegetables with the lemon juice and fresh herbs.

3. Begin steaming the salmon and the vegetables. Seven to ten minutes is enough for the lemon and the herbs to seep into the steamed content.

4. Serve hot.

Glorified Bunch of Small Potatoes

Ingredients:

- 6 ounces small potatoes

- 4 tablespoons extra virgin olive oil

- Any natural condiment of choice

Procedure:

1. Gently simmer the potatoes in water for 5-10 minutes. Drain them off afterwards. Retain the peels beforehand.

2. Heat the olive oil in a roasting tin, but not to burning levels.

3. Roast every side of the potatoes until crisp and golden brown. This will take at most 45 minutes.

4. Serve hot with the condiment of choice.

Snack and Drink Recipes

Veggie Brown Rice Sushi

Ingredients:

- 1 cup cooked brown rice

- 1 *nori* wrapper

- Any sliced or diced vegetable that can fit inside the sushi

Procedure:

1. Mold the brown rice into any shape, whether in a tube form or rolled into a ball. The important thing is that the vegetable must fit inside the sushi.

2. Wrap the *nori* wrapper around the formed brown rice.

3. Repeat steps 1 and 2 for any remaining amounts of vegetables, brown rice, and the *nori* wrapper.

Stretched Herbal Iced Tea

Ingredients:

- 1 bag herbal tea (any kind)
- 1 citrus fruit of choice (e.g. lemon or orange)
- 1 cup briskly-boiled water
- 2-3 cups lukewarm water
- Several ice cubes
- Honey, to taste

Procedure:

1. Depending on the strength of the resultant tea, submerge one teabag into briskly-boiled water.

2. Meanwhile, cut the citrus fruit of choice into slices that can be fit inside a glass.

3. Place the fruit slices into a tall glass that can accommodate at least five cups.

4. Carefully pour both the brewed tea and the lukewarm water into the tall glass at a distance of at least 12 inches from the glass. This is where the "stretched" part comes from, and one must avoid spills during the stretching process.

5. Add some dollops of honey based on the preferred amount of sweetness.

6. Finally, add the ice cubes.

Fruity Shaved Ice

Ingredients:

- 1-2 cups shaved ice
- 1/2-1 cup natural unsweetened fruit juice of any kind

Procedure:

1. Place the shaved ice in either a wide glass or a bowl.
2. Pour the unsweetened fruit juice on top of the shaved ice, and enjoy.

Note: One can replace shaved ice with shaved or crushed frozen fruit.

Chapter 5: Some Friendly Reminders

As with every other diet program on the planet, care, precise planning, patience, and perseverance must be taken to heart when undergoing the detoxification diet. Even in a short period like ten days, many things will happen. To ensure that the detox diet will become a success that will beget many more successes in the realm of the healthy lifestyle, keep the following friendly reminders in mind.

Do Not Starve

Other detox diets recommend taking only the formulas they sell themselves. Indeed, they may contain needed plant-based nourishment needed for detoxification, but the makers of those diets often forget that an imbalanced diet that is lacking in calories will prove detrimental to the body. Not only will the energy levels be depleted, but the metabolism process will also be slowed down. One unpleasant aftereffect is the tendency to eat more, especially unhealthy foods, once the diet period is over. This will make natural weight loss almost unachievable. Even worse, the lack of micronutrients in these other detox diets will lead to malnutrition that is based on micronutrient deficiency, which opens yet another floodgate of diseases. Other nasty effects of other detox crash diets include muscle degeneration, since the muscles have no source of energy to turn to, and an imbalance in blood sugar levels.

Hence, this detox diet espouses the idea that *forced starvation is absolutely prohibited.* Just eat the recommended foods at will and in good, moderated amounts.

Expect to Pee (and Poop and Sweat) a Lot

Since the detox diet enhances the body's natural detox functions, expect one undergoing the diet to pee a lot. Water, in particular, helps in flushing out toxins.

Excessive peeing not just happens when the detox diet goes overboard. Excessive sweating also happens, as well as the resultant excrement being too liquid and nasty-smelling. Peeing, pooping, and sweating too much can lead to dehydration if the amount of fluids being taken is not immediately replenished.

Dehydration is not just the depletion of the body's water, but is also the disrupted balance of fluids and electrolytes that can lead to ailments such as gastrointestinal distress, headaches, fatigue, irritability, skin irritations, circulatory problems, kidney failure, and heat stroke. Death also awaits one who is severely dehydrated.

To counteract dehydration, do not depend on fluids and fluids alone, unlike what some detox diets emphasize. Be well-balanced in both solids and liquids to avoid lost hours as a result of abnormally frequent trips to the bathroom.

Want a Colonic? No Thanks

Another form of the detox therapy involves cleansing the colon and intestines of toxins that may be released into the bloodstream. However, as demonstrated in the third chapter, there are beneficial bacteria that reside in the colon and intestines. If those bacteria are flushed out, the normal digestive process will be hampered, and the bad bacteria will have a good time releasing more toxins since their rivals are gone. The flushing out of good bacteria also results from the detox diet going beyond the recommended ten days.

Another bad effect of colon cleansing is dehydration, for the same reasons demonstrated in the previous section. Trace minerals such as potassium are also lost during the cleansing process, which contributes to dehydration. Other side effects of colon cleansing include nausea and vomiting.

Diet as an End to the Means, Not a Means to the End

People who want the figures of their dreams often forget that dieting is not really meant to immediately shed unwanted pounds. Dieting is truly meant for improved nourishment and nutrition. The notions of shedding that slab or beer belly in preparation for an event like showing off in a bikini should be disposed of. A proper mindset must be established first when doing the detox diet or any other diet for that matter.

As stated before, the detox diet being demonstrated in this book should be a transitional phase to a healthier lifestyle. Thinking in the long term when dieting is certainly better than thinking in the short term. One should remember that dieting must be an end to unhealthy habits and not a means to end that "awful" figure.

Conclusion

Thank you again for purchasing *"Detox Diet Guide: Lose Weight Quickly, Achieve Optimal Health and Feel Energized Through the 10 Day Detox"*!

I hope this book was able to help you to understand the ins and outs of the detox diet and why it is important to achieve a major change in only a short time.

Are you ready for the change? Tony Robbins says in order to create effective change, you need to start by being disgusted with where you are at. Are you disgusted with your health or body? Is it an ABSOLUTE MUST to change...not another moment? You need to feel the pain of where you are at to get the urgency to change and manifest the momentum to take action.

The next step is to consult your doctor or dietician before embarking on such a diet. And once you are given the final OK, you can then consult various more detoxification recipes based on the comprehensive list of allowable foods and drinks in this book. The recipes given in this book is just a starting point.

Finally, if you enjoyed this book, please take the time to share your thoughts and post a review on Amazon. It would be greatly appreciated!

I would love for you to share your experiences, stories and encouragements with me. My email address is

emmarosekindle@gmail.com

In addition, please remember to check out our Facebook page in order to find other resources and upcoming promotions:

https://www.facebook.com/joypublishing

With sincere thanks,

Emma Rose

Preview of "Paleo Desserts: Satisfy Your Sweet Tooth With Over 100 Quick and Easy Paleo Dessert Recipes and Paleo Baking Recipes"

Introduction

I want to thank you for purchasing the book, "Paleo Desserts: Satisfy Your Sweet Tooth With Over 100 Quick and Easy Paleo Dessert Recipes and Paleo Baking Recipes".

This book contains 100 Paleo dessert and baking recipes on how to prepare delectable desserts without sacrificing your health.

All my life I've had a sweet tooth. I would even go as far as to say that I had a sugar addiction! Over the last few years my sugar addiction got worse: I had dessert multiple times a day and every day (I guess being a Foods teacher didn't help much). I would joke with people by telling them that I had my servings of vegetables for the day in chocolate...except, I still didn't have the vegetables. It got pretty bad. I knew I hated eating that much dessert but I couldn't stop. I would eat one Ferrero Rochers and then go back for another. As I walked back to the treats, I would pass the mirror and think to myself, "I don't need to have this chocolate. But, ah, what the heck, I don't care." In the end, I'd have about 6 Ferrero Rochers in addition to the other treats I had earlier that day.

Finally, I had to take the huge tray of Ferrero Rochers to school to give to my students on Valentine's Day. There was no way I could eat the other 30 myself. Eating all this sugar caused a huge war within me. I knew that my extreme sugar eating was unhealthy for me but I didn't want to stop. I loved it too much. As a result, I wrestled between the ideal of where I wanted to be and the reality of where I was. I knew I had the discipline to say no to other things, so why couldn't I say no to chocolate?

I eventually came to the point where I was starting to get fed up with not feeling well. I had a lot of chronic pain in my neck and I was constantly tired. I knew that sugar was irritating the problem and causing inflammation in my body. At was starting to reach the breaking point. Ultimately, I chose to go off of sugar for at least three weeks to break the habit I had created for myself. It was seriously a miracle to stay consistent with my goal because I really didn't want to give up my favorite desserts.

Shortly after my decision to go off of sugar, I had a miscarriage. Experiencing the loss catapulted me into a massive journey to find health and proper nutrition. I did a live blood analysis with a naturopath to discover what was contributing to the terrible ways I was feeling. Seeing all the garbage I had in my blood forced me to go off of dairy, corn, oats, and wheat. I was left wondering, "What the heck am I going to eat? That stuff is in everything!"

Consequently, I stumbled upon the Paleo Free Diet. It was the most relevant diet to what I was trying to accomplish. I was able to find things to eat for breakfast, lunch and dinner. But desserts were a whole other story. I felt like something was missing and I couldn't put my finger on it. The best I could come up with was apple slices dipped in almond butter: hardly satisfying. Paleo desserts ended up being the by-product of my search to find something, anything that I could enjoy.

I encourage you to make that switch to healthier and happier desserts with the hundred delicious and irresistible recipes presented in this book. You don't need to follow the same extremity that I did. But if you are taking the Paleo Free Diet seriously, then you may find the same void of sweets in your life too. Cutting out all the processed foods and going back to the basics really does clear up the body and help it function better. I've seen the changes in my own life as hard as it's been to make those changes. You, too, can make the changes necessary and still have your sweets along the way!

Thank you again for purchasing this book. I hope you enjoy the recipes. Experiment with them and make substitutions to suit your needs. Please take some time to stop by and LIKE our Facebook page:

https://www.facebook.com/joypublishing

With gratitude,

Emma Rose

Chapter 1

Brief History of Paleo Free Diet

The Sweet Effects

Why do you love sweet food? Why do you crave for more of that dessert so much? Your anatomy would tell you that sweet foods would cause the release of dopamine in the part of the brain that is associated with motivation and reward. Not only that, but studies show that sweets also produce an increased level of serotonin. Serotonin gives you that feeling of happiness and wellbeing. That's why it is better to give a box of chocolates when you want the person to be in a good mood.

Unfortunately, the quote you can't have your cake and eat it too applies here. The bad effects that sugar brings are common knowledge. The number one disease is diabetes. People are aware of diabetes and its complications. That is why even when you intensely crave for that delicious dessert, you try to control your urges and settle for nothing instead. Well, that is if your self-control is in good condition. More often than not, people would rather risk the medical condition and eat that sweet thing with all their heart.

I have had many slip ups in my own life. I went two months without chocolate...can you believe it? Then Easter came. I found that if I gave myself an inch, I would take a mile. Eating chocolate quickly got out of control. I rebelled because I was strict for so long. You may find yourself in the same situation and find it hard to balance the sugar cravings. Once the sugar cravings are there, your body craves more and then a vicious cycle begins.

What is Paleo Free Diet?

Here is Paleo desserts to the rescue! You can have your cake and eat it too, literally. And not just cake only but lots more! Paleo is known by many names such as the cavemen diet, stone age diet and hunter-gatherer diet, to name a few. The concept behind this diet follows that of the Paleolithic era before the development of agriculture. This type of diet is still very young, only less than fifty years. However, more in depth researches and studies are being conducted to increase the information and knowledge on this diet.

The results of previous studies on the Paleo Free Diet reveal an improvement in health to the people involved. This is attributed to the fact that no processed foods and additives are included. Foods that were not available during the Paleolithic time such as dairy products, salt, sugar and grains are also not included in the preparation of the Paleo Free Diet. These ingredients are known to cause some of these diseases indirectly such as hypertension, diabetes, strokes, obesity and other heart problems. The same goes for the Paleo desserts. They are as delicious as the desserts that are found in the market but healthier.

You will notice that sugar shows up in the form of honey, maple syrup or chocolate. It can be argued that these sources are natural compared to the refined sugar which is a by-product of our industrialization and modern world. The history of chocolate dates back to the ancient Mayans who used the cacao pods as a form of currency. You can be the judge as to whether you want to include these foods in your diet. When it comes to chocolate, I prefer organic fair trade chocolate made from cacao powder. Cacao powder is more unrefined and unprocessed compared to cocoa powder.

There are a hundred recipes here guaranteed to satisfy your sweet tooth by using these prehistoric ingredients free of additives and processed foods. Are you ready to satisfy your cravings? Here are the simple and easy to follow recipes that you would surely fall in love with.

Check out the rest of "Paleo Desserts: Satisfy Your Sweet Tooth With Over 100 Quick and Easy Paleo Dessert Recipes and Paleo Baking Recipes" on Amazon

Or go to: http://amzn.to/1lZNcVI

Check Out My Other Books

Below you'll find some of my other books also available on Amazon and Kindle. Search for these titles on the Amazon website to find them.

Paleo Free Diet Guide for Beginners: Over 50 Paleo Free Recipes for Optimal Health & Fast Weight Loss

Paleo Desserts: Satisfy Your Sweet Tooth With Over 100 Quick & Easy Paleo Dessert Recipes & Paleo Baking Recipes

Raw Food Diet Guide: Lose Weight Quickly, Achieve Optimal Health & Feel Energized with the Raw Food Diet & Raw Food Recipes

Clean Eating Guide: Lose Weight Quickly, Achieve Optimal Health & Feel Energized with Clean Eating For Busy Families & Clean Eating Recipes

Alkaline Diet Guide: Lose Weight Quickly, Achieve Optimal Health & Feel Energized with the Alkaline Diet & Alkaline Recipes

Coconut Flour Recipes for Optimal Health & Quick Weight Loss: Gluten Free Recipes for Celiac Disease, Gluten Sensitivities & Paleo Free Diets

Almond Flour Recipes for Optimal Health & Quick Weight Loss: Gluten Free Recipes for Celiac Disease, Gluten Sensitivities & Paleo Free Diets

Wheat Free Diet for Beginners: Lose Weight Quickly, Achieve Optimal Health & Feel Energized with Gluten Free Recipes for Celiac Disease, Gluten Sensitivities & Paleo Free Diets

Detox Diet Guide: Lose Weight Quickly, Achieve Optimal Health & Feel Energized Through the 10 Day Detox

Sugar Detox Guide for Beginners: Lose Weight Quickly, Achieve Optimal Health, Feel Energized & Eliminate Sugar Cravings Naturally

Ketogenic Diet Guide for Beginners: How to Achieve Rapid Weight Loss, Optimal Health & Unstoppable Energy with Ketogenic Diet Recipes

Anti Inflammatory Diet for Beginners: Lose Weight Fast, Optimize Health, Slow Aging, Fight Inflammation, Conquer Pain & Increase Energy with the Anti Inflammation Diet Recipes

One Last Thing...

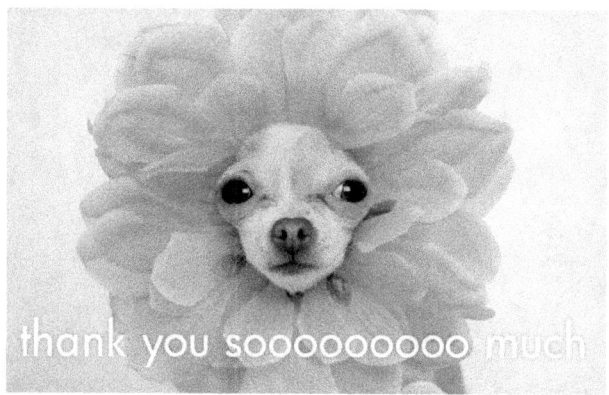

Source: Wikipedia

If you believe that this book is worth sharing, would you please take the time to let others know how it affected your life? If it turns out to make a difference in the lives of others, they will be forever grateful to you, as will I.

www.ingramcontent.com/pod-product-compliance
Lightning Source LLC
Chambersburg PA
CBHW060110300526
45791CB00018B/955